THE SECRETS OF DIABETES CODE

How to Manage Diabetes through Diet and Lifestyle

Ester M. Whicker

Copyright @2023 by Ester M. Whicker

All right reserved

No piece of this book might be duplicated, conveyed, or sent in any structure, or using all means, including copying, recording, or other electronic or mechanical strategies, without the earlier composed authorization of the publisher, with the exception of brief citations exemplified in basic audits and certain other noncommercial allowed by intellectual property regulation.

Table of Contents

Book Title
Copyright
Introduction

10. Instructions to Converse With Your Primary Care Physicians About Diabetes

Introduction

The Secrets of the Diabetes Code: How to Manage Diabetes through Diet and Lifestyle

Do you have diabetes or know someone who does? Is it safe to say that you are searching for a method for dealing with your diabetes through diet and way of life?

Given that this is valid, this book is for you. Welcome to "**The Secrets of the Diabetes Code**". This book is intended to assist you with dealing with your diabetes through diet and way of life. Inside, you'll track down data on the reasons for diabetes, as well as tips and systems for dealing with your condition.

Whether you're recently determined or have been living to have diabetes for a really long time, this book can assist you with assuming command over your wellbeing.

You'll find out about the various sorts of diabetes, as well as the job that eating regimen and exercise play in dealing with the condition. You'll likewise find the significance of stress to the executives and stay in bed keeping up with your wellbeing.

Finally, you'll learn about the most recent exploration on diabetes and what it can mean for your life. So assuming that you're prepared to assume responsibility for your wellbeing, continue to pursue. This book is your initial step headed for a better, more joyful life.

I need to begin by saying that I'm not a specialist, and this book isn't planned to supplant clinical counsel. If it's not too much trouble, counsel your PCP prior to rolling out any improvements to your eating routine or way of life. That being said, I trust this book furnishes you with significant data and systems that can assist you with carrying on with a better life. The excursion to better wellbeing begins here, with you. How about we begin!

How about we start by investigating what diabetes is. A mind boggling condition influences a huge number of individuals all over the planet. And keeping in mind that there is no fix, there are ways of overseeing it and leading a solid, satisfying life.

In this book, we'll take a gander at the various sorts of diabetes, their causes, and the effect they can have on your wellbeing.
With this information, you'll be better prepared to assume command over your condition and carry on with a day to day existence you love. So how about we begin!

There are two head sorts of diabetes: Type 1 and Type 2. Type 1 diabetes is an immune system sickness wherein the body's safe framework assaults and obliterates the cells in the pancreas that produce insulin.

Type 2 diabetes is a metabolic problem that happens when the body becomes impervious with the impacts of insulin or doesn't deliver enough of it.

The two kinds of diabetes can have serious results whenever left untreated.

In any case, with appropriate administration, individuals with diabetes can live solid, dynamic lives. So we should investigate each kind of diabetes.

The Secrets of the Diabetes Code: How to Manage Diabetes through Diet and Lifestyle. This book uncovers reality with regards to diabetes and its genuine reason, and how it very well may be relieved with basic way of life changes. It's a shrewd and extraordinary read for anybody hoping to work on their wellbeing and prosperity. So snatch a duplicate and plan to find the mysteries of the diabetes code!

In this educational book, Ester M. Whicker uncovers the genuine reason for diabetes and offers a fix that doesn't include medications or medical procedures. He shows how diabetes isn't a 'infection of glucose' yet rather a 'sickness of insulin obstruction'.

Furthermore, she gives a basic, clear arrangement that can be carried out with no medicine or intense changes to your eating routine.

The diabetes scourge is one of the greatest general wellbeing emergencies within recent memory. But, the vast majority doesn't have the foggiest idea about the genuine reason for this illness. They've been informed that it's brought about by eating a lot of sugar, or being overweight. The genuine reason for diabetes is insulin obstruction, which is brought about by various elements, including our cutting edge diet and way of life.

Fortunately there is a solution for diabetes that doesn't include medications or medical procedures. In this book, I will tell you the best way to turn around your diabetes by tending to the main driver of the issue.

By following the straightforward advances framed in this book, you can recover your wellbeing and imperativeness, and, surprisingly, switch your diabetes. You don't need to endure this illness any longer. The fix is inside your span.

This book isn't only for individuals with diabetes. Regardless of whether you're not diabetic, you can profit from the data contained in these pages. Everybody can profit from causing changes to their eating regimen and way of life to work on their wellbeing and prosperity. What's more, everybody can profit from knowing the genuine reason for diabetes, and the genuine arrangement.

The objective of this book is to furnish you with the information and instruments you really want to assume responsibility for your wellbeing. You don't need to be a casualty of diabetes. You can turn into the expert of your own fate. What's more, with this book, you will be able to roll out the improvements you want to make to work on your wellbeing and carry on with a long, blissful, and useful life.

So don't stand by one more day to begin rolling out an improvement. The ability to recuperate is in your grasp.

As you read this book, you will find out about the most recent examination on the reasons for diabetes, and how to turn it around. You will likewise find out about the strong impacts of diet and way of life on your wellbeing. You will find the significance of rest, stress the board, and exercise.

What's more, you will figure out how to establish a solid climate for you as well as your loved ones. So we should begin on the excursion to a better, more joyful life.

Now is the right time to assume back command over your wellbeing. What's more, everything begins with information. With the information contained in this book, you will actually want to settle on informed conclusions about your wellbeing and prosperity. You will be enabled to make a move and roll out the improvements you want to make.

This book isn't just about switching diabetes. It's tied in with living a long, solid, and useful life. It's tied in with feeling extraordinary consistently. It's tied in with having the energy and essentialness to do the things you love. So how about we get everything rolling on this excursion together.

I'm eager to impart this data to you, and I really want to believe that you will find it as groundbreaking as I have.

This book is only the start. There is something else to find out about wellbeing and health. Yet, with the information contained in these pages, you will have a strong groundwork on which to fabricate a sound, blissful life. So we should get everything rolling on this excursion of disclosure and recuperating. I'm eager to be your aide. Also, I anticipate catching wind of your prosperity!

Furthermore, something final: remember to partake in the excursion. Make sure to find opportunities to unwind and have some good times. Since while you're partaking in your life, you're significantly more prone to go with sound decisions.

So carve out the opportunity to do the things you love, and deal with yourself. You merit it!

I trust this book has given you the information and motivation you want to make a better life. In any case, information alone isn't sufficient. You additionally need to make a move.

So I urge you to begin little and roll out each improvement in turn. Also, as you see the positive aftereffects of your endeavours, you'll be propelled to roll out considerably more improvements. In what would seem like no time, you'll be carrying on with the existence you've for practically forever cared about!

Assuming that you have any inquiries or need extra assets, kindly make it a point to out. I'm here to assist in any capacity I can with canning.
Likewise, I'd really like to hear from you about your experience.

I trust you've viewed this book as supportive and enlightening. I anticipate hearing from you and aiding you on your excursion to better wellbeing!

Meanwhile, make sure to deal with yourself. Practice good eating habits, move your body, and partake in the straightforward things throughout everyday life. Furthermore, make sure to grin. Since when you grin, you feel improved, yet you likewise cheer others up. So go out there and spread some euphoria and bliss!

Also, one final piece of insight: take things each day in turn. Rome wasn't underlying a day, nor is a solid, cheerful life. So centre around the current second and do all that can be expected with what you have. Furthermore, believe that, after some time, the easily overlooked details you truly do consistently will amount to large outcomes. So partake in the excursion, and trust the cycle!

Also, presently, my last words to you: much thanks to you. Much obliged to you for setting aside some margin to pursue this book.

I trust you've thought that it is useful and moving. Also, I need to say thank you for being you.

You are an extraordinary and exceptional individual, and the world is a superior spot since you're in it. So continue to be you, and keep on spreading your light. The world requires more individuals like you!

Furthermore, I want you to enjoy all that life has to offer on your excursion to better wellbeing and bliss. What's more, recall: you have this!
On the off chance that you or a friend or family member has diabetes, I urge you to get this book. It's loaded with significant data and bits of knowledge that can assist you with assuming command over your condition and have a solid, blissful existence. The information you'll acquire from this book can be the way to carrying on with your best life. Wait don't as well - get your duplicate today! You'll be happy you did.

Chapter One
What is Diabetes Code?

The "diabetes code" is a term that alludes to the complicated connection between hereditary qualities, climate, and way of life factors that add to the improvement of diabetes. It's imagined that a blend of these variables would be able to "code" or trigger the beginning of diabetes. This code is special for every person; it's actually being contemplated and perceived by researchers.

Notwithstanding hereditary qualities and climate, there are different elements that can add to the diabetes code.

These include:

- Corpulence and weight gain

- An unfortunate eating routine

- Absence of actual work

- Stress

- Rest issues

- The presence of other ailments, similar to hypertension or elevated cholesterol

- The utilization of specific meds, similar to steroids

- Openness to specific natural poisons
These are only a portion of the elements that can be important for the diabetes code.

We should discuss the job of corpulence and weight gain in the diabetes code. Stoutness is a gamble factor for diabetes, and overabundance of muscle to fat ratio can influence how well your body utilizes insulin. This can prompt insulin opposition, which is vital consider the improvement of diabetes. Shedding pounds and keeping a solid weight can assist with bringing down your gamble of creating diabetes.

Rudiments of Diabetes Code

The following are several critical rudiments of the diabetes code:

- Hereditary qualities assume a part in the improvement of diabetes.

- Stoutness is a significant gambling factor for diabetes.

- Way of life factors, similar to eating less and work out, can influence your gamble of diabetes.

- Overseeing pressure and getting sufficient rest can likewise assist with lessening your gamble of diabetes.

- Overseeing other ailments, similar to hypertension and elevated cholesterol can likewise lessen your gamble of diabetes.

- Certain prescriptions, similar to steroids, can build your gamble of creating diabetes.

- Diabetes can altogether affect your personal satisfaction.

- Individuals with diabetes have a higher gamble of creating other medical issues, similar to coronary illness and stroke.

- There are different types of diabetes, which include type 1, type 2, and gestational diabetes.

Facts

- Individuals with diabetes can deal with their condition with way of life changes, prescription, and different medicines.

- A solid eating regimen is a significant piece of diabetes for the executives.

- Getting customary active work is likewise a significant piece of diabetes for the executives.

Here is the following bunch of essentials:

- Blood glucose observing is a significant piece of diabetes, the executives.

- Blood glucose levels can be made with drug and way of life changes.

- There are various sorts of blood glucose observing gadgets accessible.

- Understanding what various food sources mean for blood glucose levels is significant.

- Liquor utilization can influence blood glucose levels.

- Stress of the executives is a significant piece of diabetes the board.

- Despondency is more normal in individuals with diabetes.

Here are the following 10 fundamentals:

- Certain ailments, similar to rest apnea, can influence blood glucose levels.

- A few meds can influence blood glucose levels.

- Ordinary exams with your primary care physician are significant.

- Certain individuals with diabetes require insulin treatment.
- There are various sorts of insulin treatments.

- There are potential confusions related to diabetes.

- Pregnancy can influence diabetes.

- Pregnant ladies with diabetes have a higher gamble of inconveniences.

- Kids with diabetes require unique consideration and checking.

What it means for the body

Here are ways diabetes can influence the body:

- Diabetes can harm the veins.

- Diabetes can harm the nerves.

- Diabetes can harm the eyes.

- Diabetes can harm the kidneys.

- Diabetes can harm the skin.

- Diabetes can harm the heart.

- Diabetes can harm the mouth.

- Diabetes can harm the feet.

- Diabetes can influence the mind.

- Diabetes can influence sexual capability.

- Diabetes can influence rest.
- Diabetes can cause weight gain or misfortune.

- Diabetes can influence temperament and conduct.

- Diabetes can cause different side effects.

- High blood glucose levels can cause lack of hydration.

- High blood glucose levels can cause the development of ketones.

- Low blood glucose levels can cause side effects like insecurity and uneasiness.

- Low blood glucose levels can be perilous whenever left untreated.

- Low blood glucose levels can cause hypoglycemic trance-like state.

- Diabetic ketoacidosis is a possibly dangerous complexity.

- Hyperosmolar hyperglycemic state is a difficult condition that can happen in individuals with diabetes.

Here's more data about diabetes:

- Individuals with diabetes might encounter inconveniences that aren't straightforwardly connected with blood glucose levels.

- Individuals with diabetes have an expanded gamble of disease.

- Individuals with diabetes have an expanded gamble of creating osteoporosis.

- Individuals with diabetes have an expanded gamble of gum infection.

- Individuals with diabetes have an expanded gamble of hearing misfortune.

- Individuals with diabetes have an expanded gamble of sadness.

- Individuals with diabetes have an expanded gamble of nervousness.

- Individuals with diabetes have an expanded gamble of dietary issues.

Diabetes complexities? Realities for you:

- Individuals with diabetes have an expanded gamble of foot issues.

- Individuals with diabetes have an expanded gamble of skin issues.

- Individuals with diabetes have an expanded gamble of eye issues.

- Individuals with diabetes have an expanded gamble of dental issues.

- Individuals with diabetes have an expanded gamble of hearing misfortune.

- Individuals with diabetes have an expanded gamble of Alzheimer's sickness.

- Individuals with diabetes have an expanded gamble of pancreatic disease.

- Individuals with diabetes have an expanded gamble of cardiovascular illness.

Ways it tends to be analyze

Here are ways diabetes can be analyzed:

- A fasting blood glucose test can be utilized to analyze diabetes.

- An irregular blood glucose test can be utilized to analyze diabetes.

- An oral glucose resilience test can be utilized to analyze diabetes.

- A hemoglobin A1c test can be utilized to analyze diabetes.

- A pee test can be utilized to analyze diabetes.

- An actual assessment can be utilized to analyze diabetes.

- A clinical history can be utilized to analyze diabetes.

- A family background of diabetes can be utilized to analyze diabetes.

More ways diabetes can be analyzed

- Research center tests can be utilized to analyze diabetes.

- An eye assessment can be utilized to analyze diabetes.

- A foot assessment can be utilized to analyze diabetes.

- A dental assessment can be utilized to analyze diabetes.

- An assessment of the sensory system can be utilized to analyze diabetes.

- An assessment of the kidneys can be utilized to analyze diabetes.

- An assessment of the heart can be utilized to analyze diabetes.

- An assessment of the lungs can be utilized to analyze diabetes.

Here is the following arrangement of data:

- A rest study can be utilized to analyze diabetes.

- A chest X-beam can be utilized to analyze diabetes.

- An electrocardiogram (EKG) can be utilized to analyze diabetes.

- An echocardiogram can be utilized to analyze diabetes.

- A Holter screen can be utilized to analyze diabetes.

- A pressure test can be utilized to analyze diabetes.

- A blood vessel ultrasound can be utilized to analyze diabetes.

- A coronary angiogram can be utilized to analyze diabetes.

More ways diabetes can be analyzed:

- A barium swallow test can be utilized to analyze diabetes.

- A CT sweep can be utilized to analyze diabetes.

- An attractive reverberation imaging (X-ray) sweep can be utilized to analyze diabetes.

- A positron emission tomography (PET) output can be utilized to analyze diabetes.

- A liver capability test can be utilized to analyze diabetes.

- A blood coagulation test can be utilized to analyze diabetes.

- A total blood count (CBC) can be utilized to analyze diabetes.

Kinds of Diabetes

There are three principal sorts of diabetes:

- Type 1 diabetes is a safe framework ailment.

- Type 2 diabetes is a metabolic problem.

- Gestational diabetes is a brief type of diabetes that happens during pregnancy.

Each kind of diabetes is unique and requires various medicines.

Type 1 diabetes is an immune system illness, and that implies the body's resistant framework erroneously goes after the insulin-creating cells in the pancreas.

This prompts a lack of insulin, which thus causes high blood glucose levels. Type 1 diabetes is normally analyzed in kids and youthful grown-ups, yet it can happen at whatever stage in life.

Individuals with type 1 diabetes need to take insulin infusions to deal with their blood glucose levels. Without insulin, they can turn out to be extremely wiped out and try to bite the dust.

Side effects

Symptoms of the Type1 diabetes

Normal side effects of type 1 diabetes for you:

- Inordinate thirst.

- Regular pee.

- Outrageous craving.

- Unexplained weight reduction.

- Exhaustion.

- Hazy vision.

- Slow-recuperating wounds.

- Successive contaminations.

- Fruity-smelling breath.

- Stomach torment.

- Sluggishness or disarray.

- Abrupt mind-set changes.

- Abrupt character changes.

I can give more detail on these side effects. The initial not many side effects I recorded are the most widely recognized, and are known as the "three Ps" of diabetes: polydipsia (unnecessary thirst), polyuria (successive pee), and polyphagia (outrageous craving).

These side effects happen in light of the fact that the body can't involve glucose for energy, so it goes to fat and muscle all things being equal. This can prompt weight reduction and shortcoming. Foggy vision and deafness or shivering in the hands and feet are other normal side effects.

Causes

Reasons for the Type 1 Diabetes

Here are the best reasons for type 1 diabetes:

- Family ancestry.

- Hereditary vulnerability.

- Openness to certain infections.

- Immune system response.

- Natural variables.

- Lack of vitamin D.

- Low birth weight.

- Insulin opposition.

- Celiac infection.

- Eating handled food varieties.

- Lack of sleep.

- Openness to synthetics.

- Corpulence.

- Stress.

- Contamination.

- Type 1 diabetes can likewise happen immediately.

More data on these causes

How about we start with family ancestry. On the off chance that an individual has a parent or kin with type 1 diabetes, they are at a higher gamble of fostering the actual condition.

Also, certain hereditary markers have been related with type 1 diabetes, so individuals with these markers might be bound to foster the condition. Openness to certain infections, like Coxsackie B infection and cytomegalovirus, has additionally been connected to type 1 diabetes.

Finding

Ways type 1 diabetes can be analyzed

Here are normal strategies used to analyze type 1 diabetes:

- Blood glucose test.

- A1C test.

- Glucose resilience test.

- Oral glucose resistance test.

- Pee test.

- C-peptide test.

- Immune response test.

- Islet cell neutralizer test.

- Insulin autoantibody test.

- Thyroid capability test.

These are only a couple of the tests that can be utilized to analyze type 1 diabetes. Could you like me more about any of these?

How about we start with the blood glucose test. This is one of the most widely recognized tests used to analyze type 1 diabetes. A blood test is taken and broken down to gauge how much glucose in the blood. An individual with type 1 diabetes will regularly have elevated degrees of glucose in their blood. Notwithstanding a blood glucose test, an individual's A1C levels are likewise tried. A1C is an estimation of normal blood glucose levels over a few months. An individual with type 1 diabetes will normally have a high A1C level.

I can tell you more about the glucose resistance test, which is one more typical test used to analyze type 1 diabetes. This test includes drinking a sweet fluid that contains glucose. The individual's blood glucose levels are then estimated at explicit spans throughout the following couple of hours. An individual with type 1 diabetes will regularly have a postponed reaction to the glucose drink, and their blood glucose levels will stay high even after the test is finished.

Treatment

Ways type 1 diabetes can be dealt with

Treatment for type 1 diabetes commonly includes a blend of way of life changes and medicine. I'll begin by making sense of the way of life changes:

- Eating a sound, adjusted diet.

- Getting standard activity.

- Overseeing feelings of anxiety.

- Keeping a solid weight.

- Checking blood glucose levels.

- Taking insulin infusions or utilizing an insulin siphon.

- Utilizing a constant glucose screen.

- Getting customary clinical exams.

- Having this season's virus chance and different inoculations as suggested by a specialist.

There are a few unique kinds of prescription that can be utilized to treat type 1 diabetes. The most well-known kind of medicine is insulin. There are a few distinct kinds of insulin, including quick acting, short-acting, moderate acting, and long-acting.

Each sort of insulin has an alternate span of activity and is utilized at various times. Notwithstanding insulin, there are additionally oral drugs that can be utilized to treat type 1 diabetes. These incorporate sulfonylureas, meglitinides, and alpha-glucosidase inhibitors.

Anticipation

Ways type 1 diabetes can be forestalled

While there is no reliable method for forestalling type 1 diabetes, there are a few things that might assist with lessening the gamble. These include:

- Breastfeeding babies.

- Keeping away from openness to certain infections.

- Postponing the presentation of strong food varieties for babies.

- Keeping a solid weight.

- Getting standard activity.

- Eating a sound eating regimen.

- Taking specific nutrients and enhancements.

- Keeping away from specific synthetic compounds and pesticides.

- Keeping up with great rest propensities.

- Getting standard clinical tests.

- Monitoring the early signs and side effects of type 1 diabetes.

More Avoidance Techniques

The following are a couple of more counteraction techniques:

- Restricting openness to air contamination.

- Rehearsing great cleanliness.

- Diminishing pressure.

- Restricting openness to electromagnetic fields.

- Keeping a sound stomach microbiome.

- Staying away from specific meds that might build the gamble of type 1 diabetes.

It's essential to take note that not these avoidance procedures have been experimentally demonstrated to lessen the gamble of type 1 diabetes. Nonetheless, they might merit considering assuming you are worried about your gamble.

Here are other interesting points with regards to forestalling type 1 diabetes:

- Getting hereditary testing to recognize hereditary gamble factors.

- Grasping the admonition of type 1 diabetes in youngsters.

- Early finding and treatment of type 1 diabetes.

- Family backing and training.
- Diabetes research and clinical preliminaries.

Additionally significant some gamble factors for type 1 diabetes, similar to hereditary qualities, are beyond our control. Notwithstanding, we can in any case do whatever it takes to decrease our gamble by going with sound way of life decisions.

What is type 2 diabetes?

Type 2 diabetes is one more kind of diabetes that is very not quite the same as type 1 diabetes. In type 2 diabetes, the body either doesn't make sufficient insulin or can't utilize the insulin it makes appropriately. This is called insulin opposition. Insulin obstruction can cause blood glucose levels to rise, which can prompt serious medical issues over the long haul.

Some gambling factors for type 2 diabetes include being overweight or corpulent, having a family background of diabetes, and driving a stationary way of life. Type 2 diabetes is more normal than type 1 diabetes, and it can happen at whatever stage in life.

There are a few unique ways type 2 diabetes can be dealt with. The initial step is much of the time making way of life changes, such as eating a sound eating routine, getting customary activity, and shedding pounds if necessary.

There are likewise a few unique kinds of prescriptions that can be utilized to treat type 2 diabetes, including metformin, sulfonylureas, and GLP-1 receptor agonists. At times, insulin treatment may likewise be required. There is no one size-fits-all way to deal with treating type 2 diabetes, and the best treatment plan will change from one individual to another.

Side effects

The following are a couple of ordinary symptoms of type 2 diabetes:

- Expanded thirst.

- Expanded hunger.

- Weight reduction, regardless of whether you are eating more than expected.

- Sleepiness.

- Hazy vision.

- Injuries or contaminants that don't recuperate.

- Unexplained weight gain.

- Unexplained balding.

- Dim patches of skin.

- Feeling extremely powerless or tired.

- Feeling peevish.

- Feeling extremely parched.

- Peeing frequently.

There are a couple of different side effects of type 2 diabetes that are more uncommon yet worth monitoring. These include:

- Tingling.

- Night sweats.

- Sexual brokenness.

- Cerebral pains.

- Skin rashes.

- Gastrointestinal issues.

- Ulcer.

- Back torment.

- Temperament changes.

- Fever.

- Dry mouth.

- Muscle torment.

On the off chance that you are encountering any of these side effects, seeing a doctor is significant.

Reasons for type 2 diabetes

There are a wide range of reasons for type 2 diabetes, and generally a blend of elements lead to the improvement of the condition. Here are likely causes:

- Hereditary qualities.

- Age.

- Being overweight or corpulent.

- Inactive way of life.

- Eating an eating routine high in sugar and refined starches.

- Drinking sweet refreshments.

- Elevated degrees of stress.

- Absence of rest.

- Hypertension.

- Elevated cholesterol levels.

- Low degrees of active work.

- Aggravation.

- Insulin opposition.

The following are a couple of additional reasons for type 2 diabetes:

- Smoking.

- Openness to ecological poisons.

- Certain meds like steroids or antipsychotics.

- History of gestational diabetes.

- Polycystic ovary disorder (PCOS).

- Fundamental immune system conditions.

- Certain persistent diseases.

- Pregnancy.

- Injury, like a physical issue or medical procedure.

- Cytomegalovirus (CMV) contamination.

- HIV contamination.

- Synthetic openness.

- Utilization of specific chemicals.

- Utilization of some antipsychotic drugs.

Conclusion

I really want 15 different ways type 2 diabetes can be analyzed.

Most well known ways that type 2 diabetes is analyzed. These include:

- Fasting blood glucose test.

- Arbitrary blood glucose test.

- HbA1c test.

- Oral glucose resistance test.

- Glycated egg whites (GA) test.

- C-peptide test.

- Insulin autoantibody test.

- Free unsaturated fat test.

- Oral glucose resistance test utilizing a nonstop glucose screen.

- Glycated hemoglobin A1C and albuminuria test.

There are a few other more uncommon ways that type 2 diabetes can analyzed, include:

- Exogenous insulin reaction test.
- Insulin discharge test.

- Oral glucagon feeling test.

- Intravenous glucose resilience test.

- Pancreatic beta cell capability test.

- Islet cell capability test.

- Islet cell neutralizer test.

- Immunohistochemistry.

- Proinsulin reaction test.

- First stage insulin emission test.

These tests might be utilized in specific circumstances, for example, assuming that you are pregnant or have other fundamental medical issues.

Treatment

Ways type 2 can be dealt with

Here are the familiar ways that type 2 diabetes is dealt with

- Way of life changes, like eating a solid eating regimen and practicing routinely.

- Drugs, like metformin, insulin, and GLP-1 agonists.

- Blood glucose checking.

- Insulin siphon treatment.

- Insulin pens or needles.

- Ceaseless glucose screens.

- Careful medicines, like gastric detour or sleeve gastrectomy.

- Weight reduction medical procedure.

- Bariatric medical procedure.

- Way of life the executives programs.

The following are a couple of greater treatment choices for type 2 diabetes:

- Dietary directing.

- Self-observing of blood glucose levels.

- Patient instruction.

- Individualized care plans.

- Practice programs.

- Stress the board.

- Psychosocial support.

- Care based pressure decreases.

- Mental social treatment.

- Bunch treatment.

- Conduct weights the executive programs.

- Vascular medical procedure.

- Vascular stents.

- Angioplasty.

These are only a couple of the numerous treatment choices accessible for type 2 diabetes.

Avoidance

Ways it tends to be forestalled

The following are 15 methods for decreasing your gamble of creating type 2 diabetes:

- Keep a sound weight.

- Work-out routinely.

- Follow a sound eating routine.

- Stop smoking.

- Diminish pressure.

- Get sufficient rest.

- Keep away from exorbitant liquor utilization.

- Stay away from sweet beverages.

- Eliminate handled food sources.

- Eat a lot of fiber.

- Eat more leafy foods.

- Control circulatory strain and cholesterol.

- Know your family ancestry.

- Get tested for prediabetes.

Instructions to lessen the gamble of Diabetes

Here are an additional ways of diminishing your gamble of creating type 2 diabetes:

- Take diabetes avoidance classes.

- Keep your blood glucose levels in a sound reach.

- Oversee other ailments.

- Look for help for psychological well-being conditions.

- Use alerts with specific drugs.

- Receive any available immunization shots.

- Take a diabetes counteraction program.

- Know about natural poisons.

- Get evaluated for diabetes during pregnancy.

- Keep a solid body weight prior to getting pregnant.

- See a specialist consistently.

What is gestational diabetes?

Gestational diabetes is a sort of diabetes that can happen during pregnancy.

During pregnancy, the placenta produces chemicals that can prompt insulin obstruction. This implies that the body's cells don't answer insulin as well as they ought to.

Gestational diabetes normally disappears after the child is conceived, yet it can prompt medical conditions for both the mother and the child. Ladies who have gestational diabetes have a higher gamble of creating type 2 diabetes further down the road.

I can give more detail. Gestational diabetes is many times analyzed through a glucose resilience test. This test estimates your blood glucose levels when you drink a glucose-rich beverage. The test is commonly given somewhere in the range of 24 and 28 weeks of pregnancy.

In the event that you have gestational diabetes, your PCP will suggest a treatment plan. This might incorporate making sound way of life changes, like eating a solid eating routine and practicing consistently.

Now and again, you might have to take insulin or different drugs to control your blood glucose levels.

Side effects

The most well-known side effects of gestational diabetes include:

- Expanded thirst.

- Expanded hunger.

- Exhaustion.

- Queasiness.

- Regular pee.

- Dry mouth.

- Obscured vision.

- Slow-recuperating wounds.

- Unexpected weight gain.

- Bothersome skin.

- Vaginal or skin contaminations.

-   Unreasonable   perspiring,   particularly   around evening time.

- Expanding in the hands or feet.

- Aggravation of the gums.

Notwithstanding the side effects I recently recorded, you may likewise insight:

- Unsteadiness.

- Cerebral pains.

- Shivering or deadness in the hands or feet.

- Shivering or deadness around the mouth.

- Desires for sweet food sources.

- Stomach torment.

- Languor.

- Sluggishness.

- Crabbiness.

- Regurgitating.

- Trouble relaxing.

- Leg cramps.

- Unexplained weight reduction.

- Loss of cognizance.

Causes

A few normal reasons for gestational diabetes include:

- Family background of diabetes.

- Corpulence.

- Absence of actual work.

- Race or nationality.

- Hypertension.

- Polycystic ovary disorder.

- Age (the gamble of creating gestational diabetes increments with age).

- Elevated degrees of amniotic liquid.

- Various pregnancies (twins, trios, and so on.).

- History of unsuccessful laborers.

- Diabetes during a past pregnancy.

There are a couple of extra causes that I can fill you in about. For instance, a mother's weight and body shape can assume a part in the improvement of gestational diabetes. Additionally, some exploration recommends that pressure and sorrow might expand the gamble of creating gestational diabetes.

At long last, disease, aggravation, and the utilization of specific prescriptions during pregnancy may likewise expand the gamble. Obviously, there are different elements that might build the gamble of creating gestational diabetes. A medical care supplier can assist you with understanding the particular gamble factors that concern you.

Inconveniences

Absolutely! I can likewise give you some data on the potential confusions of gestational diabetes. These include:

- Macrosomia (child is bigger than typical).
- Shoulder dystocia (when the child's shoulder stalls out during birth).

- Hypoglycemia (low glucose) in the child.

- Jaundice (yellowish skin or eyes).
- Respiratory pain condition (a breathing issue).

- Hypocalcemia (low degrees of calcium in the blood).

- Hypomagnesemia (low degrees of magnesium in the blood).

Finding

Ways gestational diabetes can be analyzed

There are various ways gestational diabetes can analyzed, include:

- Glucose challenge test.

- Glucose resilience test.

- Arbitrary blood glucose test.

- Glycated hemoglobin test.

- Insulin challenge test.

- Fasting blood glucose test.

- Oral glucose resistance test.

- C-peptide test.

- Glycosylated serum protein test.

- Development of the child.

- Ultrasound of the child.

- Actual assessment.

- Clinical history.

Certainly! I can give more data on a portion of these tests. For instance, the glucose challenge test is a typical evaluating test for gestational diabetes. It includes drinking a sweet fluid and afterward having your blood drawn an hour after the fact. On the off chance that the blood glucose level is high, you might have to take a glucose resilience test. This test is like the glucose challenge test, however it includes drinking a sweet fluid and having your blood drawn consistently for three hours.

Treatment

Ways gestational diabetes can be dealt with

Totally! Gestational diabetes can be treated with different strategies, including:

- Dietary changes.

- Work out.

- Insulin treatment.

- Metformin treatment.

- Glucose observing.

- Self-checking of blood glucose.

- Pre-birth care.

- Post pregnancy care.

- Breastfeeding.

- Weight the executives.

- Mental directing.

- Stress the board.

- Conduct directing.

- Perinatal schooling classes.

- Assumption directing.

- Pre-pregnancy advising.

I can carefully describe a portion of these medicines, on the off chance that you'd like. For instance, dietary changes might include diminishing how much carbs and refined sugars are in your eating regimen.

Customary activity is likewise significant, as it assists the body with utilizing insulin all the more successfully.

Insulin treatment might be essential in the event that dietary changes and exercise are sufficiently not to control blood glucose levels. With insulin treatment, you should screen your blood glucose levels all the more intently and change your insulin portion depending on the situation.

There are multiple ways of diminishing your gamble of creating gestational diabetes. They include:

- Keeping a sound weight.

- Eating a sound eating regimen.

- Getting normal actual work.

- Not smoking.

- Overseeing pressure.

- Getting sufficient rest.

- Overseeing pulse.

- Overseeing cholesterol levels.

- Lessening openness to poisons.

- Abstaining from smoking, liquor, and road drugs.

- Keeping away from unreasonable weight gain during pregnancy.

- Overseeing previous ailments.

- Family arranging.

- Hereditary directing.

- Pre-birth care.

I might want to expand more on the significance of keeping a sound weight. Overabundance of body weight is a significant gambling factor for creating gestational diabetes.

This is on the grounds that an abundance of fat tissue can deliver chemicals that impede the body's capacity to appropriately utilize insulin.

Thus, keeping a sound load previously and during pregnancy can assist with lessening the gamble of creating gestational diabetes. A solid eating routine is likewise significant, as it can assist with managing glucose levels and backing generally wellbeing. Normal actual work can likewise assist with holding blood glucose levels under wraps and decrease pressure.

We should discuss smart dieting. Eating a fair eating regimen is critical to forestalling gestational diabetes. The right equilibrium of carbs, proteins, and fats can assist with keeping up with stable blood glucose levels. Eating more fiber and less refined starches can likewise help.

Fiber dials back the processing and ingestion of starches, which can assist with controlling blood glucose levels.

It is additionally vital to stay away from handled and sweet food sources, as they can cause spikes in blood glucose levels. Drinking a lot of water is likewise significant, as it helps flush overabundance of glucose out of the body.

Chapter Two
Way of life Changes That Work on Your Diabetes

One significant way of life change is to get sufficient activity. Standard active work can assist with further developing blood glucose control, increment insulin awareness, and decrease pressure. Hold back nothing 150 minutes of moderate-power active work every week.

It's additionally vital to get sufficient rest, as absence of rest can influence blood glucose levels. Stressing the board is one more significant part of diabetes for the executives. Persistent pressure can make it more challenging to control blood glucose levels.

Attempting pressure decreases methods like yoga, reflection, or profound relaxation. In conclusion, assuming that you smoke, stopping can assist with bringing down your gamble of diabetes-related entanglements.

We should discuss taking care of one practice that can assist you with remaining sound. Rehearsing taking care of oneself is significant for everybody, except its particularly significant for individuals with diabetes.

Taking care of oneself can incorporate things like overseeing pressure, getting normal actual work, and eating a solid eating regimen. Taking care of oneself additionally incorporates dealing with your profound wellbeing. This can incorporate things like rehearsing care, journaling, or associating with others. Dealing with your profound wellbeing can assist you with better adapting to the difficulties of living with diabetes.

There are additionally unambiguous taking care of oneself practices for blood glucose the executives.

In the first place, testing your blood glucose levels routinely is vital.

This will assist you with recognizing designs in your glucose levels and make acclimations to your eating regimen and work-out routine appropriately.

Second, keeping a food diary can assist you with following what you're eating and what it means for your glucose levels.

Third, accepting your drugs as endorsed by your doctor is significant.

Ultimately, it is vital to be ready for crises. Keep a unit with your glucose meter, drugs, and snacks in the event that your glucose levels become shaky.

Presently we should discuss medicine adherence. Taking your drugs precisely as recommended by your PCP is vital for diabetes. It's likewise vital to converse with your PCP about any progressions in your wellbeing, including assuming you're feeling unwell or encountering any aftereffects from your drug.

In the event that you're experiencing difficulty accepting your medicine as endorsed, converse with your PCP about methodologies to further develop your drug adherence. For instance, you could set updates on your telephone, utilize a pillbox, or ask a relative or companion to assist you with recollecting.

We should discuss smart dieting propensities. Eating a solid, adjusted diet is significant for diabetes, the executives. Here are a few explicit tips:

- Pick entire grains over refined grains.

- Pick products of the soil over handled food sources.

- Pick lean proteins, like fish, poultry, and plant-based proteins.

- Limit added sugars and sweet beverages.

- Limit soaked and trans fats.

- Peruse food marks and pick food sources with the least measure of added sugars and sodium.

- Hold back on the eating plan, and try not to skip dinners.

We should continue on toward solid cooking tips. Cooking at home can assist you with controlling your part estimates and pick better fixings. Here are some cooking tips:

- Utilize different flavours and spices to add flavour to your food, rather than adding salt.

- Have a go at cooking techniques that don't need added fats, like barbecuing, simmering, or steaming.

- Pick heart-solid oils, like olive oil, avocado oil, and canola oil.

- Eat the rainbow by including various leafy foods of various tones.

Presently we should discuss feast arranging. Feast arranging is a significant piece of diabetes on the board. It can assist you with adhering to a solid eating regimen and control your piece sizes. Here are a few hints for feast arranging:

- Plan your feasts for the week early.

- Cook additional servings of quality dinners and store them in the refrigerator or cooler for some other time.

- Pre-slash foods grown from the ground so they're prepared to eat when you're ravenous.

- Pack solid snacks for when you're in a hurry.

We should discuss going with sound decisions while feasting out. Feasting out can be quite difficult when you have diabetes, however it doesn't need to be. Here are a few hints:

- Pick dishes that are steamed, barbecued, or heated rather than broiled.

- Request dishes with vegetables and entire grains.

- Stay away from huge segments by sharing dishes or requesting a hors d'oeuvre rather than an entrée.

- Stay away from sweet beverages and pick water or unsweetened chilled tea.

We should discuss the significance of active work. Active work is a significant piece of diabetes on the board. It can assist you with controlling your blood glucose levels and work on your general wellbeing.

The CDC suggests that grown-ups with diabetes get something like 150 minutes of moderate-force high-impact action every week.

You can likewise include some muscle-reinforcing exercises at least two days of the week.

Take a stab at separating your action into 10-minute pieces over the course of the day in the event that you're experiencing difficulty squeezing it into your timetable.

We should examine a few explicit kinds of active work that are great for individuals with diabetes. Strolling is an incredible choice since it's not difficult to do and requires no unique hardware.

Swimming is another great decision since it's delicate on your joints. Cycling, yoga, and moving are great choices also. In the event that you experience difficulty with versatility, seat practices are a decent choice. Jujitsu is another choice that is particularly great for further developing equilibrium and forestalling falls. Anything you pick, ensure it's something you appreciate and can stay with over the long haul.

Presently we should discuss a few hindrances to actual work and how to conquer them. One normal hindrance is an absence of time.

Assuming you're in a rush, have a go at separating your action into short blasts over the course of the day. For instance, you could go for a 10-minute stroll during your mid-day break or stroll up the steps as opposed to taking the lift.

Assuming you're experiencing difficulty finding inspiration, take a stab at defining objectives and remunerating yourself for contacting them. Or on the other hand, track down a companion or relative to practice with to make it more tomfoolery. Another normal hindrance is joint agony. Attempt low-influence exercises like swimming or water heart stimulating exercise.

I'm happy you're so intrigued! I have something else for you about unambiguous medical advantages of actual work for individuals with diabetes. Actual work can assist with bringing down blood glucose levels and further develop glucose control. It can likewise work on your rest, lessen pressure, and increment your energy levels.

Furthermore, actual work can further develop your pulse, cholesterol levels, and body weight. It can likewise bring down your gamble of creating other persistent sicknesses, like coronary illness and stroke. Furthermore, it could work on your psychological wellness and temperament. The best part is that active work is free and requires no extraordinary gear.

We should discuss the gamble of injury. While active work is ok for the vast majority, keeping some wellbeing guidelines is significant. To begin with, gradually and steadily increment your movement level over the long haul.

Then, pick exercises that are suitable for your wellness level and state of being. Likewise, make certain to heat up and chill off appropriately. Furthermore, assuming you experience any aggravation or distress, pause and look for clinical counsel.

In the event that you have a specific medical issue, similar to coronary illness or hypertension, check with your PCP prior to beginning another action.

I need to stress the significance of consistency. Perhaps the most ideal option for your wellbeing is to be genuinely dynamic consistently. Attempt to find a movement that you appreciate and can stay with over the long haul.

Begin with something you realize you can resolve, regardless of whether it's only 10 minutes per day. Whenever you've laid out a daily schedule, you can slowly build the length and force of your exercises. Keep in mind, any movement is superior to no action by any means. So get out there and get rolling!

Chapter Three
The Job of Meds in Treating Diabetes

There are a wide range of sorts of prescriptions that can be utilized to treat diabetes. The most well-known ones are called oral hypoglycemic specialists. These incorporate metformin, sulfonylureas, thiazolidinediones, meglitinides, and dipeptidyl peptidase-4 (DPP-4) inhibitors. There are additionally injectable drugs, for example, insulin, glucagon-like peptide-1 (GLP-1) agonists, and amylin analogs. Every medicine works another way to bring down blood glucose levels.

For example, metformin is the most ordinarily recommended medicine for diabetes. It works by bringing down how much glucose that your liver makes and expanding the awareness of your phones to insulin.

Sulfonylureas assist your pancreas with making more insulin. Thiazolidinediones assist with making your cells more delicate to insulin. Meglitinides animate your pancreas to deliver more insulin. DPP-4 inhibitors delay the breakdown of GLP-1, which assists your pancreas with making more insulin.

There's even more! Insulin is a chemical that assists control with blood glucose levels. It very well may be infused or taken through an insulin syphon. GLP-1 agonists work by animating the pancreas to make more insulin and dialing back absorption.

Amylin analogs work by dialing back absorption and diminishing how much glucose is delivered by the liver. These are only a portion of the numerous prescriptions that can be utilized to treat diabetes. It's critical to converse with your primary care physician about which prescription is ideal for you. They will consider your singular necessities and inclinations while making a proposal.

Something significant to recollect is that drugs are just important for the treatment plan for diabetes. A solid way of life is likewise vital to dealing with the condition. This incorporates eating a reasonable eating regimen, remaining truly dynamic, and checking your blood glucose levels routinely.

Prescription ought to be utilized related to these different parts of treatment for the best outcomes. You and your PCP will cooperate to make a customized plan that accommodates your singular necessities.

I can likewise educate you concerning mix treatment, which is when at least two prescriptions are utilized together to treat diabetes. This should be possible for various reasons, for example, in the event that a solitary medicine isn't controlling blood glucose levels or on the other hand in the event that the results of a solitary drug are excessively extreme. There are a few distinct blends of drugs that can be utilized, and your primary care physician will suggest the best one for you.

These can incorporate blends of oral prescriptions, infusions, and other treatment choices.

One more point connected with meds is the issue of adherence. Adherence alludes to how intently an individual follows their medicine routine. This is a significant thought, as non-adherence can prompt unfortunate diabetes control and entanglements.

A portion of the explanations behind non-adherence incorporate neglecting to take prescription, trouble bearing the cost of drugs, or encountering secondary effects. Assuming you are experiencing difficulty sticking to your drug routine, converse with your PCP about ways of moving along. This could incorporate setting updates, utilizing pillboxes, or tracking down monetary help.

A connected subject is medicine security. It's critical to know about the expected symptoms of any drug you're taking. This is particularly valid for individuals with diabetes, as certain prescriptions can cause hypoglycemia (low blood glucose).

The most well-known symptoms of diabetes meds incorporate gastrointestinal bombshell, cerebral pain, and skin rashes.

In the event that you experience any secondary effects, converse with your primary care physician immediately. They might have the option to recommend an elective medicine that won't cause similar incidental effects. It's additionally critical to keep all of your medical services suppliers informed about any prescriptions you're taking, including non-prescription drugs and enhancements.

We should discuss drug adherence and cost. As referenced, the expense of drugs can be a boundary to adherence. Yet, there are a few projects that can assist with making meds more reasonable. For instance, numerous drug stores offer rebate cards or coupons for physician recommended meds.

There are additionally quiet help programs presented by drug organizations, as well as taxpayer supported initiatives like Federal health insurance Part D. Your PCP or drug specialist can give more data about these projects. You can likewise converse with a social specialist or caseworker at your medical care supplier's office for help.

There are additionally a few general tips that can assist with making your drugs more reasonable. For instance, you can inquire as to whether there is a nonexclusive rendition of your medicine that is more affordable. You can likewise inquire as to whether there are any coupons or markdown programs accessible for your medicine.

Furthermore, you can look around at changed drug stores to track down the best cost. A few drug stores, similar to those at big box stores, may offer lower costs on meds. Lastly, remember to check with your insurance agency to check whether your drug is covered.

Notwithstanding the expense of meds, there are additionally different expenses related with overseeing diabetes. These incorporate the expense of clinical supplies, for example, test strips and lancets, as well as the expense of specialist's visits and lab tests. On the off chance that you're attempting to bear the cost of these expenses, there are a couple of choices accessible.

In the first place, check with your insurance agency to check whether any of these expenses are covered. Second, there are a few associations that offer monetary help for clinical supplies. Lastly, some local area wellbeing focuses give minimal expense or free clinical consideration, including diabetes care.

I might want to zero in on the social and close to home parts of residing with diabetes. It's normal for individuals with diabetes to encounter sensations of uneasiness, misery, and stress.

These sentiments can be because of the actual difficulties of overseeing diabetes, as well as the social disgrace and separation that individuals with diabetes at times face.

Assuming you're encountering these sentiments, it means quite a bit to connect for help. Converse with your PCP, family, and companions about the thing you're going through. You can likewise look for help from a psychological wellness proficient, like a specialist or instructor.

There are additionally a few things you can do all alone to deal with the social and inner difficulties of diabetes. One accommodating methodology is classified as "self-empathy." This includes being thoughtful and understanding towards yourself, as opposed to thumping yourself when things aren't working out positively.

It's likewise essential to find an encouraging group of people or individuals who comprehend what you're going through.

This can incorporate joining a diabetes support bunch, either face to face or on the web. Lastly, remember to reserve a margin for yourself to unwind and do things you appreciate. This can assist with decreasing pressure and further develop your general prosperity.

Dealing with your psychological wellness by rehearsing great rest hygiene is likewise significant. Getting sufficient quality rest is significant for overseeing diabetes. This implies hitting the hay and awakening simultaneously consistently, keeping away from screens before sleep time, and establishing an agreeable rest climate.

Moreover, you can rehearse unwinding strategies, like profound breathing, moderate muscle unwinding, or reflection. Finding an opportunity to unwind can help you rest better and deal with your diabetes all the more really.

There's something else to examine! Another tip is to zero in on the things you have some control over, as opposed to the things you can't. For instance, you have no control over your family ancestry or the manner in which others treat you, yet you have some control over how you deal with yourself.

Attempt to zero in on the positive parts of living with diabetes, for example, the way that you're giving a valiant effort to deal with the condition. This can assist you with feeling more enabled and in charge of your wellbeing. Moreover, you can utilize an everyday organizer or diary to follow your triumphs and achievements.

To wrap things up, I might want to underline the significance of keeping an inspirational perspective. It's not difficult to get deterred and feel overpowered while living with diabetes.

However, it's memorable and vital that you're giving a valiant effort and you're in good company.

Encircle yourself with individuals who support you, and advise yourself that you can deal with this. Lastly, deal with your physical and emotional wellness by getting sufficient rest, working out, eating great, and rehearsing self-empathy.

Chapter Four
The Advantages of Self Administration for Diabetes

Self-administration is a vital part of diabetes care. It's that you play a functioning job in dealing with your condition, as opposed to depending entirely on your PCP or other medical care experts.

Self-administration incorporates things like checking your glucose routinely, accepting meds as endorsed, eating a sound eating regimen, and getting normal activity.

It likewise incorporates finding out about your condition and tracking down ways of adapting to the pressure of living with diabetes. The advantages of self-administration incorporate better glucose control, worked on generally wellbeing, and a more noteworthy feeling of strengthening.

One of the main advantages of self-administration is better glucose control. This is on the grounds that you're playing a functioning job in observing your glucose and making changes to your eating regimen and way of life depending on the situation.

By keeping your glucose inside a sound reach, you can stay away from inconveniences like kidney illness, coronary illness, and nerve harm.

Furthermore, self-administration can assist you with feeling more in charge of your wellbeing and lead to work on by and large wellbeing. You might have more energy, less nervousness, and a more uplifting perspective on life.

We should discuss the mental advantages of self-administration. Self-administration can fundamentally affect your psychological wellness. At the point when you're effectively engaged with your diabetes care, you might feel less worried, restless, or discouraged.

This is on the grounds that you're assuming responsibility for your condition and giving your best to stay sound. Self-administration can likewise assist you with feeling more sure and fit for taking care of difficulties that come your direction.

Also, it can assist you with feeling more associated with others and less disconnected. These advantages can prompt superior personal satisfaction.

We should discuss how self-administration can assist you with your connections. Self-administration can emphatically affect your associations with loved ones. At the point when you're effectively associated with your diabetes care, you might feel more sure and less restless, which can make it simpler to interface with others.

Furthermore, you might have the option to converse with your friends and family all the more straightforwardly about your condition, which can encourage a feeling of trust and closeness.

This thus can prompt more strong and sound connections. Furthermore, obviously, this can decidedly affect your general prosperity.

How about we examine the effect of self-administration on your public activity. Self-administration can assist you with remaining dynamic and engaged with your local area. For instance, you might feel more propelled to go to get-togethers or join clubs and associations. This is on the grounds that you're feeling far improved genuinely and inwardly, and you have a feeling of direction and association.

Associating with others is significant for your general prosperity, and self-administration can assist you with doing that all the more really. Also, self-administration can give you the certainty to attempt new things and meet new individuals.

We can likewise discuss the monetary advantages of self-administration.

While diabetes can be costly, self-administration can assist you with setting aside cash over the long haul. This is on the grounds that you might have the option to forestall or defer diabetes entanglements, which can be exorbitant to treat. For instance, self-administration might assist you with keeping away from the requirement for dialysis or a kidney relocation, the two of which are over the top expensive techniques.

Also, you might have the option to diminish your requirement for medicine or other medical care administrations. Thus, while self-administration requires a little speculation of time and exertion, it can eventually set aside your cash.

We should discuss the drawn out advantages of self-administration. Self-administration can prompt superior wellbeing and prosperity temporarily, yet additionally in the long haul.

For instance, self-administration can assist you with staying away from the improvement of long haul diabetes entanglements, for example, nerve harm, kidney illness, coronary illness, and eye issues.

Moreover, it can assist you with keeping a solid weight, which is related with better well being and life span. Eventually, the advantages of self-administration are combined and can intensify over the long run, prompting a more drawn out, better, and seriously satisfying life.

One region we haven't discussed at this point is the significance of self-administration for your work life. Self-administration can assist you with being more useful and effective at work. At the point when you feel great truly and inwardly, you're better ready to concentrate and finish things.

Also, self-administration can assist you with trying not to put a hold on from work because of sickness or other well being related issues.

Over the long haul, this can prompt more prominent work fulfillment and vocation achievement. In this way, by putting resources into self-administration, you're putting resources into your future.

We should discuss how self-administration can work on your associations with medical care suppliers. At the point when you're effectively engaged with your diabetes care, you're bound to have a positive relationship with your PCP, diabetes instructor, and other medical services suppliers.

This is on the grounds that you're playing a functioning job in your consideration and working with them collectively. A decent connection with your medical services suppliers can prompt better correspondence, more precise findings, and better therapy results. At last, this can prompt better general wellbeing and prosperity.

A few hints on the best way to begin with self-administration. One of the initial steps is to set little, reachable objectives.

These could be things like following your blood glucose levels or eating better feasts.

Whenever you've accomplished these objectives, you can define additional difficult objectives over the long run. Another tip is to track down an emotionally supportive network, like family, companions, or a care group. Having individuals who get it and support you can have a significant effect in your excursion. At last, show restraint toward yourself and celebrate even little triumphs en route.

There are numerous self-administration apparatuses and assets accessible to help you on your excursion. One model is a diabetes board application. These applications can assist you with following your blood glucose levels, drug use, and the sky's the limit from there.

There are additionally numerous internet based networks and gatherings where you can interface with other people who are likewise overseeing diabetes.

Furthermore, your neighborhood library or medical clinic might have assets, for example, diabetes, board classes or care groups. Also, obviously, you can constantly connect with your medical care group for guidance and backing.

I'll share a few normal difficulties with self-administration. One test is remaining propelled. This can be troublesome when you don't see prompt outcomes or when you experience misfortunes. Another test is using time productively.

Carving out the opportunity to squeeze self-administration into your bustling timetable can be intense. Lastly, dealing with feelings is another normal test. Diabetes can be sincerely depleting, and it's not unexpected to have promising and less promising times. Notwithstanding, it means quite a bit to track down solid ways of adapting to these feelings.

There are multiple ways of beating these difficulties. One way is to zero in on the "why" behind your objectives. Help yourself to remember the justifications for why you're dealing with your diabetes, for example, to feel significantly improved, to carry on with a more extended life, or to set a genuine model for your friends and family.

Another tip is to separate your objectives into little, reasonable advances. For instance, rather than expecting to shed 20 pounds, take a stab at planning to lose a couple of pounds each week. This will cause your objective to feel more attainable and less overpowering.

There are a few procedures for remaining inspired. One system is to compensate yourself for meeting your objectives. This could be something as straightforward as scrubbing down or indulging yourself with an extraordinary dinner. Another system is to find a responsible accomplice.

This could be a companion, relative, or another person who is likewise overseeing diabetes. Having somebody to check in with and share your headway can have a major effect. At long last, make sure to celebrate even little victories. These can be a wellspring of inspiration while you're feeling deterred.

I need to leave you with a message of trust and consolation. Overseeing diabetes is an excursion, and it's generally expected to have highs and lows. In any case, with the right devices and procedures, you can have an effect on your wellbeing and personal satisfaction.

Furthermore, recollect that, you're in good company on this excursion - there are numerous other people who are additionally overseeing diabetes. By making little strides and praising your triumphs, you can have a major effect in your life. Good luck on your excursion to better wellbeing!

Chapter Five
Diminishing the Gamble of Entanglements from Diabetes

There are numerous ways of diminishing the gamble of entanglements from diabetes. One is to monitor your blood glucose levels. This should be possible by taking drugs, following a sound eating regimen, and practicing routinely.

One more method for diminishing the gamble of confusions is to keep your pulse and cholesterol levels taken care of. This should be possible by taking drugs, following a sound eating regimen, and practicing routinely. Finally, it's critical to have normal check-ups with your primary care physician to distinguish any issues from the beginning.

As well as dealing with your blood glucose, circulatory strain, and cholesterol levels, there are different advances you can take to decrease your gamble of confusions.

One is to stop smoking, assuming you smoke right now. Smoking builds the gamble of numerous medical conditions, including coronary illness and stroke. Another significant step is to deal with your feelings of anxiety.

Stress can adversely affect your general wellbeing and can make it harder to deal with your diabetes. Unwinding methods like yoga and reflection can be useful in decreasing pressure. Lastly, make a point to get sufficient rest. Unfortunate rest can likewise build your gamble of inconveniences.

There are numerous alternate ways of remaining solid and diminish your gamble of entanglements, even past what we've proactively talked about.

For instance, you can make a point to receive an immunization shot against sicknesses like this season's virus and pneumonia.

These diseases can be more serious for individuals with diabetes. Moreover, make a point to wear shoes that fit well and have great help to stay away from foot issues. Lastly, deal with your teeth and gums by cleaning and flossing consistently. Unfortunate oral wellbeing has been connected to an expanded gamble of diabetes-related complexities.

Focusing on your emotional wellness is additionally significant. Diabetes can negatively affect your psychological prosperity, and it's critical to resolve any issues you might have. In the event that you're feeling discouraged or restless, converse with your primary care physician or an emotional wellness proficient.

They can assist you with tracking down ways of adapting and work on your personal satisfaction.

Lastly, make sure to carve out a margin for yourself. Taking care of oneself is significant, and it can incorporate things like having some time off from your everyday schedule, carving out opportunities to unwind, and doing things you appreciate.

I realize I've provided you with a great deal of data, yet there are still a few additional things I might want to specify. In the first place, make a point to remain informed about your condition.

There are numerous assets accessible to assist you with finding out about diabetes, including books, sites, and care groups. The more you are familiar with your condition, the better you'll have the option to oversee it. Living with diabetes can be testing, and it's essential to give yourself credit for the headway you're making.

As well as dealing with your physical and emotional wellness, you can likewise do whatever it takes to work on your monetary wellbeing.

Overseeing diabetes can be costly, and it means quite a bit to track down ways of diminishing expenses. One method for doing this is to converse with your primary care physician about less expensive options in contrast to your ongoing meds.

You can likewise ask your insurance agency in the event that there are any limits accessible for diabetes-related supplies. Likewise, there are numerous associations that offer monetary help for individuals with diabetes. You can likewise check with your nearby public venue or clinic for assets.

At last, I might want to address something frequently neglected with regards to diabetes: your otherworldly wellbeing. Living with diabetes can be an otherworldly test, and it means quite a bit to track down ways of interfacing with your confidence or convictions.

This can assist you with tracking down importance and reason in your life, even notwithstanding difficulty.

You can do this by rehearsing supplication, reflection, or investing energy in nature. Anything you pick, the significant thing is to find something that assists you with associating with an option that could be greater than yourself.

One more significant part of overseeing diabetes is social help. Social help is the help you get from companions, family, and local area individuals. Research has demonstrated the way that social help can assist with further developing blood glucose levels and personal satisfaction.

It's critical to construct areas of strength for an organization that you can depend on for help. There are numerous ways of doing this, including joining a care group, making new companions, or contacting lifelong companions. What's more, remember to give as well as get social help - you can help other people by being a listening ear or a shoulder to rest on.

At last, I might want to discuss ways of life changes that can assist with working on your personal satisfaction. Rolling out little improvements to your regular routine can have a major effect by the way you feel. For instance, you can attempt to get more actual work by going for a day to day stroll or joining a rec centre.

You can likewise work on your eating regimen by adding more products of the soil and eliminating handled food varieties. Furthermore, remember to carve out a margin for yourself to do things you appreciate, such as perusing, playing an instrument, or painting. Carving out an opportunity to unwind and re-energize is significant for your general wellbeing.

One way of life change that is frequently neglected is the significance of rest. Getting sufficient rest is pivotal for individuals with diabetes, as it can assist with further developing blood glucose levels and lessen pressure. It's suggested that grown-ups get 7-8 hours of rest each evening.

To work on your rest, you can take a stab at heading to sleep and awakening simultaneously consistently, keeping away from screens before bed, and keeping your room cool and dull. In the event that you're experiencing difficulty dozing, it means quite a bit to converse with your PCP or a rest subject matter expert.

A last way of life change that can further develop your wellbeing is figuring out how to oversee pressure. Stress can adversely affect blood glucose levels, so it means a lot to track down ways of unwinding and de-stress. Some pressure decrease procedures incorporate profound breathing, yoga, or reflection.

You can likewise take a stab at journaling, investing energy in nature, or tracking down an imaginative source for your pressure. What's more, make sure to enjoy reprieves over the course of the day, regardless of whether it's only for a couple of moments. Finding an opportunity to re-energize can assist you with feeling more loose and centred.

Something last I might want to make reference to is the significance of self-support. Self-support implies supporting yourself and it is addressed to ensure your requirements. This is particularly significant with regards to your medical care.

You can advocate for yourself by clarifying some things, doing your own exploration, and ensuring you comprehend your treatment plan. It's likewise critical to find a medical services group that you trust and feel OK with. Self-promotion can have a major effect in your general personal satisfaction.

Presently I might want to discuss the significance of defining objectives.

Defining objectives is a significant piece of self-administration. It assists you with remaining persuaded and provides you with a feeling of achievement when you arrive at your objectives. There are one or two sorts of objectives you can set.

One is a Savvy objective, which represents Explicit, Quantifiable, Feasible, Pertinent, and Time-bound. An illustration of a shrewd objective may be "I will walk 30 minutes every day for the following month". One more kind of objective is a cycle objective, which is centred on the interaction instead of the result.

An illustration of a cycle objective may be "I will find 10 minutes every day to sit and unwind". At long last, there are result objectives, which are centred on the outcome. An illustration of a result objective may be "I will shed 5 pounds in the following 2 months".

It's critical to have a blend of various sorts of objectives, and to define objectives that are significant to you. Make sure to fire a little and develop over the long run. Also, remember to commend your victories, regardless of how enormous or little they are.

Lastly, I might want to discuss the significance of remaining positive. It's not difficult to get hindered by the negative parts of diabetes, however zeroing in on the positive also is significant. There are numerous things to be thankful for, even amidst a difficult circumstance.

One method for remaining positive is to rehearse appreciation; by thinking about the things you're thankful for every day. You can likewise attempt positive confirmations, which are articulations you rehash to yourself to significantly impact your outlook.

One more method for remaining positive is to search for the silver linings in tough spots. For instance, assuming you need to change your eating regimen, you could find that you feel more empowered and amazing.

Furthermore, assuming you possess more energy for taking care of one, you could find that your connections get to the next level. At long last, remember to chuckle! Giggling is an incredible pressure reliever, and it can likewise support your safe framework and decrease irritation. So remember to track down the humour throughout everyday life, even in tough spots.

One more significant piece of remaining positive is self-sympathy. This implies being caring and understanding towards yourself, in any event, when you commit errors.

The fact that everyone commits errors makes it not difficult to be challenging for ourselves, however it memorable essential.

At the point when you commit an error, attempt to be delicate with yourself and gain from the experience. Also, recall that, you're in good company - there are numerous others going through exactly the same thing. By rehearsing self-empathy, you can remain positive and zeroed in on your objectives.

In conclusion, it's critical to find a local area of individuals who comprehend what you're going through. This can be a care group, a web-based local area, or basically a companion or relative who is there for you. Having a strong local area can have a major effect by the way you feel, and it can likewise give useful assistance and exhortation. Keep in mind; you don't need to go through this by itself.

Chapter Six
The Monetary Weight of Diabetes

The monetary weight of diabetes is a genuine and huge issue for some individuals. The expenses of diabetes incorporate the expense of drug and supplies, yet additionally the expense of specialist's visits, lab tests, and other medical care administrations.

Furthermore, individuals with diabetes frequently need to miss work because of their condition, which can prompt lost compensation. The all out cost of diabetes is assessed to be more than $300 billion every year in the US alone. This cost isn't just a weight on people, yet in addition to the medical care framework and society overall.

One method for diminishing the monetary weight of diabetes is to attempt to forestall it in any case. This should be possible through way of life changes like eating a sound eating routine, practicing consistently, and keeping a solid weight.

Again, ordinary check-ups and screenings can assist with getting diabetes right on time, before it prompts exorbitant complexities. Assuming you have diabetes, it's likewise essential to work with your medical care group to successfully deal with your condition. This can assist with forestalling exorbitant confusions and work on your personal satisfaction.

One more method for diminishing the monetary weight of diabetes is to ensure you're benefiting from your protection inclusion. Converse with your insurance agency about what's covered, and ensure you're exploiting every one of the advantages accessible to you.

You may likewise be qualified for government help programs that can assist with counterbalancing the expense of diabetes. Moreover, numerous drug organizations offer help projects to assist with taking care of the expense of meds. Get some information about these projects and whether you may be qualified.

Additionally, there are various ways of lessening your personal expenses for diabetes supplies and meds. One choice is to utilize mail-request drug stores, which frequently offer limits on diabetes supplies. You can likewise get some information about conventional renditions of prescriptions, which are frequently more affordable than brand-name drugs.

Lastly, there are various coupons and rebate programs accessible for diabetes supplies and meds. A large number of these projects are offered straight by the makers, so it merits really looking at their sites for more data.

Notwithstanding the monetary weight, diabetes can likewise have a critical profound cost. Dealing with your profound wellbeing as well as your actual health is significant.

There are numerous assets accessible to assist you with adapting to the personal difficulties of diabetes.

These incorporate care groups, advising, and stress the board strategies. It's likewise essential to carve out opportunities for charming exercises, like leisure activities, investing energy with loved ones, and dealing with yourself. Setting aside a few minutes for taking care of oneself isn't childish, yet fundamental to keeping up with your wellbeing.

On the off chance that you're a parental figure for somebody with diabetes, dealing with your own requirements too is significant. Parental figure burnout is a genuine concern, and setting aside a few minutes for you is significant.

There are various care groups and different assets accessible for guardians of individuals with diabetes. You may likewise need to consider rest care, which is a break from your providing care obligations. Dealing with yourself isn't just significant for your own wellbeing, yet it will likewise assist you with being a superior guardian.

It's likewise essential to be familiar with diabetes-related lawful issues. Individuals with diabetes might confront various lawful difficulties, for example, protection inclusion issues, separation in the working environment, and end-of-life choices.

It's critical to know about your privileges and to look for legitimate assistance if necessary. There are various associations that furnish lawful help to individuals with diabetes, for example, the American Diabetes Affiliation and the Handicap Privileges Training and Guard Asset.

Lastly, it's essential to know about the most recent diabetes research. New medicines and advances are being fostered constantly, and it's critical to remain informed about what's accessible.

This might incorporate new prescriptions, insulin siphons, ceaseless glucose screens, and that's just the beginning. Assuming that you're keen on partaking in clinical preliminaries, you can track down data on clinicaltrials.gov.

This site is an asset for individuals who need to find out about and partake in clinical preliminaries.

On the off chance that you have diabetes, it's additionally critical to know about your freedoms with regards to travel. The Air Transporter Access Act safeguards the privileges of individuals with handicaps while going via air.

This incorporates the option to convey diabetes supplies and drugs on board the plane, as well as the option to demand help from carrier staff.

What's more, numerous carriers have programs that give extraordinary help to individuals with diabetes. It means quite a bit to contact your carrier early on to find out about their strategies and to make any important plans.

Chapter Seven
The Diabetes and Your
Psychological well-being

Psychological well-being is a vital piece of living with diabetes. Many individuals with diabetes experience some type of sadness or uneasiness sooner or later. This is much of the time connected with the pressure of living with persistent sickness, as well as the physical and close to home cost of diabetes.

Gloom and tension can likewise make it harder to oversee diabetes and can build the gamble of diabetes-related complexities.

It's essential to know about the indications of sadness and uneasiness, and to look for help if necessary. There are various medicines that can be successful, including treatment, drug, and way of life changes.

Mental conduct treatment (CBT) is one of the best medicines for gloom and tension in individuals with diabetes. CBT is a sort of talk treatment that assists individuals with recognizing and changing negative idea examples and ways of behaving. It tends to be done separately or in a social scene, and it's typically a present moment.

CBT has been displayed to further develop blood glucose control, diminish diabetes-related trouble, and work on personal satisfaction. There are likewise various self improvement devices in view of CBT rules that can be utilized to oversee discouragement and nervousness.

One more typical worry for individuals with diabetes will be diabetes-related trouble, otherwise called diabetes burnout. This is a condition of physical, close to home, and mental weariness that can result from the pressure of residing with diabetes.

Diabetes-related pain can prompt issues with diabetes on the board, for example, skipping insulin dosages or not following a solid eating routine. It's essential to know about the indications of diabetes-related trouble, for example, feeling overpowered, furious, or liable. On the off chance that you're encountering these side effects, it means quite a bit to contact your medical services group for help.

Taking care of oneself is a significant piece of diabetes for the executives, both for your physical and psychological well-being. Taking care of oneself can be separated into three principal classifications: physical, close to home, and profound. Actual taking care of oneself incorporates exercises like working out, eating a solid eating regimen, and getting sufficient rest.

Profound taking care of oneself can incorporate investing energy with loved ones, doing things you appreciate, and figuring out how to oversee pressure.

Otherworldly taking care of oneself can incorporate exercises like reflection, petition, or going to strict administrations. Working on something for yourself consistently, regardless of how little, can have a major effect in your general prosperity.

Social help is one more significant part of taking care of oneself for individuals with diabetes. Having areas of strength for an organization can assist with decreasing pressure, increment inspiration, and work on personal satisfaction.

There are various ways of building major areas of strength for an organization. This can incorporate joining a care group, chipping in, or basically trying to invest more energy with loved ones.

Having only one individual to converse with and trust in can have a major effect. Keep in mind, even little thoughtful gestures from others can hugely affect your temperament.

While taking care of oneself is significant, being benevolent to you is additionally significant. Self-sympathy is a vital piece of overseeing diabetes. This implies being caring and understanding towards yourself, in any event, when you commit errors or feel like you're not working really hard.

Whipping yourself or having a blameworthy outlook on your diabetes will just exacerbate the situation. So all things considered, attempt to show restraint, acknowledge your sentiments, and spotlight on giving your all. Keep in mind; you're working effectively by simply dealing with your diabetes consistently.

Finally, setting aside a few minutes for fun is significant. Having a great time isn't just great for you're close to home prosperity, however it can likewise assist you with staying with your diabetes the board plan.

Doing things you appreciate can give you something to anticipate and can assist you with adapting to pressure.

This could be anything from heading out to the motion pictures, taking a class, or simply investing energy with companions. It's vital to find something that makes you cheerful and to set aside a few minutes for it, regardless of whether it's only for a couple of moments every day.

As well as setting aside a few minutes for entertainment only, it means quite a bit to giggle. Giggling isn't just great for your mind-set, yet it can likewise decidedly affect your actual wellbeing. Giggling has been displayed to bring down pulse, further develop rest quality, and lift the resistant framework.

It's likewise been displayed to deliver endorphins, which can decrease torment and further develop temperament. So feel free to chuckle, whether it's watching a parody or simply telling a wisecrack with a companion. Your body and psyche will thank you for it!

Something different that might help is participating in exercises that advance care. Care is the act of living right now without judgment. This should be possible through things like reflection, yoga, or even going for a stroll and focusing on your environmental elements.

Care can assist with decreasing pressure, increment centre, and further develop mind-set. So make time to dial back and spotlight on the current second, regardless of whether it's only for a couple of moments every day. You might find that it has a major effect.

In conclusion, remember to rehearse appreciation. Appreciation is the demonstration of being grateful and valuing what you have in your life. This should be possible by writing in an appreciation diary, telling somebody you're thankful for them, or just pondering the beneficial things in your day to day existence.

Appreciation has been displayed to increment satisfaction, further develop rest, and lessen side effects of sorrow. In this way, regardless of whether you're having a hard day, pause for a minute to ponder the things you're thankful for. It might assist with placing things in context.

Part of carrying on with a sound existence with diabetes is figuring out how to deal with your pressure. Stress can hugely affect your diabetes, so it means quite a bit to track down ways of overseeing it.

One methodology is to recognize the wellsprings of stress in your life and attempt to track down ways of lessening or kill them. This could mean defining limits with others, expressing no to additional obligations, or setting aside a few minutes for you. It means a lot to track down solid ways of adapting to pressure, like working out, journaling, or conversing with a companion.

One more significant part of overseeing diabetes is defining objectives that are explicit, quantifiable, and reachable. Having explicit objectives assists you with zeroing in on what you need to accomplish and keeping tabs on your development.

Quantifiable objectives permit you to keep tabs on your development and perceive that you are so near accomplishing your objective.

Furthermore, ensuring your objectives are reachable guarantees that you're not getting yourself in a position for disappointment. For instance, rather than laying out an objective to run a long distance race, you could lay out an objective to run a 5K race inside a specific measure of time.

While laying out objectives for your diabetes the executives, taking into account the idea of Brilliant goals is likewise significant. Savvy is an abbreviation that represents explicit, quantifiable, achievable, important, and time-bound.

This implies that your objectives ought to be explicit, have a quantifiable result, be feasible inside a sensible time period, be pertinent to your general diabetes the board, and have an unmistakable cutoff time.

For instance, a Savvy objective may be to decrease your glucose levels by 10 in no less than a half year by practicing three times each week and eating a better eating regimen.

One more significant piece of objective lying out is separating your objectives into more modest, reasonable advances. This is known as lumping. Separating a bigger objective into more modest undertakings can cause it to feel more reasonable and assist you with remaining persuaded.

For instance, in the event that you want to get more fit, you could piece it down into more modest objectives like shedding two pounds every month, strolling for 30 minutes per day, and eating a reasonable eating routine.

Each time you arrive at a more modest objective, you'll feel a feeling of achievement that will assist with keeping you spurred.

A supportive method for remaining focused with your diabetes the board objectives is to utilize a prizes framework. This is an approach to rousing yourself by compensating yourself for arriving at your objectives.

For instance, you could compensate yourself with a back rub or another set of shoes after you arrive at a specific achievement in your diabetes. Or on the other hand you could indulge yourself with a pleasant feast following seven days of adhering to your good dieting plan. The key is to pick remunerations that are significant to you and that will assist you with remaining persuaded.

As well as defining objectives and utilizing a prizes framework, one more significant piece of diabetes the executives are tracking down ways of partaking in the excursion.

It's not difficult to become involved with zeroing in on the ultimate objective and neglect to partake all the while. Yet, it's memorable critical that diabetes the board is a long lasting excursion, and it's OK to require your investment and commend the little triumphs en route.

You could partake in the process by tracking down ways of making good dieting fun and pleasant or by setting up a steady climate for yourself.

A critical piece of partaking in the excursion of diabetes the executives is tracking down ways of praising yourself. This could mean commending your advancement by journaling, enjoying some time off, or indulging yourself with something you appreciate.

It's likewise essential to praise yourself for your identity personally, not only for your diabetes the executives. You could commend your assets, values, and achievements. Tracking down ways of cherishing and value yourself can assist you with remaining propelled on your diabetes the board venture.

It's additionally essential to make sure to pardon yourself on the off chance that you don't generally meet your objectives. It's normal to have promising and less promising times in your diabetes. At the point when you have a mishap, attempt to gain from it and continue on.

Thrashing yourself over errors will just make it harder to refocus. All things being equal centre around what you can do another way sometime later. What's more, recollecting your value as an individual isn't characterized by your diabetes, the executives. You are more than your diabetes.

While you're on your diabetes board venture, it's additionally critical to ensure you're dealing with your psychological well-being.

Emotional wellness is similarly essentially as significant as actual wellbeing, and it's critical to resolve any issues you may have. This could incorporate conversing with a specialist, getting sufficient rest, and rehearsing unwinding procedures.

Dealing with your emotional wellness can assist you with dealing with your diabetes all the more really and work on your general personal satisfaction.

A piece of your emotional wellness excursion could likewise incorporate figuring out how to reevaluate pessimistic contemplations. This is the most common way of distinguishing negative idea examples and supplanting them with additional positive and reasonable ones.

For instance, in the event that you're feeling overpowered by your diabetes the board, you could see yourself, "I can't deal with this." A more supportive idea may be, "I can deal with this slowly and deliberately."

Figuring out how to rethink negative contemplations can take time and practice, yet it tends to be exceptionally useful in working on your psychological wellness.

One more significant piece of dealing with your diabetes is figuring out how to manage troublesome feelings. While you're feeling worried, baffled, or irate, it tends to be enticing to attempt to stay away from those sentiments.

Nonetheless, this frequently exacerbates them. All things considered, attempt to permit yourself to feel your sentiments. You could have a go at rehearsing care or breathing activities to assist you with managing troublesome feelings.

What's more, recollect, it's alright to request help from others on the off chance that you're battling to adapt. Your companions, family, and medical care group are there to help you.

Finally, remember to deal with your actual wellbeing also. It's not difficult to become involved with dealing with your diabetes; however it's vital to ensure you're dealing with your general wellbeing. This incorporates getting normal exams, eating a solid eating regimen, and getting sufficient activity.

Dealing with your actual wellbeing can assist with further developing your glucose levels, decrease pressure, and further develop your general prosperity. Furthermore, recall, taking care of oneself isn't childish - it's fundamental for dealing with your diabetes.

Chapter Eight
The Social Shame of Diabetes

One part of living with diabetes that can be hard to oversee is the social shame that can accompany it. Certain individuals actually have the misinterpretation that diabetes is brought about by private shortcoming or an absence of resolve. This can prompt sensations of disgrace or shame, which can make it harder to discuss diabetes and look for help.

Nonetheless, it's memorable vital that diabetes is an ailment, not an individual fizzling. Nothing remains to be embarrassed about, and there are many individuals who comprehend what you're going through.

One more part of the social shame of diabetes is that finding a steady environment can be hard.

It's not generally simple to find individuals who comprehend what you're going through. In any case, there are various care groups accessible for individuals with diabetes.

These gatherings can be an extraordinary spot to track down figuring out, data, and backing. There are additionally online networks where you can interface with other people who have diabetes.

The American Diabetes Affiliation has a site where you can find nearby care groups and an internet based discussion where you can interface with others.

The social shame of diabetes can likewise cause it hard to feel sure about yourself. It's not difficult to feel like you're not adequate or that you can't do things the manner in which you used to. In any case, it's memorable vital that you are as yet unchanged individual you were before your determination. Diabetes is a piece of your life, yet it doesn't need to characterize you.

You can in any case seek after your objectives and partake in your life. It's generally expected to have promising and less promising times in your diabetes the board, yet don't allow that to characterize your self-esteem.

There are various procedures you can use to deal with the social disgrace of diabetes. One is to instruct you about diabetes and be ready to address questions. Having the right data can give you the certainty to discuss your condition. It can likewise be useful to interface with other people who have diabetes.

This can provide you with a feeling of local area and backing. At last, attempt to zero in on the things you have some control over, similar to your own mentality and activities. By zeroing in on what you can do, you can feel more in charge of your diabetes and your life.

It's likewise critical to recollect that the social shame of diabetes can adversely affect your emotional wellness. At times, it can prompt misery or nervousness. On the off chance that you're battling with your emotional wellness, it means quite a bit to connect for help.

There are various assets accessible, including guiding, treatment, and drugs. Dealing with your psychological well-being is similarly just about as significant as dealing with your actual wellbeing. It's anything but an indication of a shortcoming to look for help - it's an indication of solidarity.

At long last, it's memorable vital that the social shame of diabetes isn't just about you - it's about everybody. By attempting to decrease the shame, you can assist with establishing a steadier climate for individuals with diabetes.

This can incorporate revolting against your experience, upholding for change, and teaching others about diabetes. Indeed, even little activities can have a major effect.

Together, we can attempt to make an existence where diabetes is acknowledged and perceived.

For a bigger scope, support can assume a significant part in decreasing the social disgrace of diabetes. Promotion can take many structures, incorporating partaking in research, bringing issues to light, and making some noise about the requirements of individuals with diabetes. There are various associations that promoter for individuals with diabetes, for example, the

American Diabetes Affiliation and JDRF. These associations work to work on the existences of individuals with diabetes through exploration, training, and backing. You can get involved by supporting these associations, sharing their work, or partaking in their occasions.

While decreasing the social disgrace of diabetes is significant, it's not by any means the only method for working on your personal satisfaction.

Taking care of oneself is a fundamental piece of dealing with your diabetes. This incorporates dealing with your actual wellbeing, yet it additionally incorporates dealing with your psychological and profound wellbeing.

Carving out margin for yourself, defining limits, and focusing on your requirements are immensely significant parts of taking care of oneself. At the point when you deal with yourself, you're better ready to deal with others and carry on with a full and satisfying life.

As well as dealing with yourself, it's vital to construct serious areas of strength for an organization. This can incorporate family, companions, and, surprisingly, online networks. Having an encouraging group of people can assist you with feeling not so much confined but rather more associated.

Your encouraging group of people can offer profound help, functional help, and, surprisingly, a listening ear.

You can likewise be a wellspring of help for other people, which can assist you with feeling more deliberate and associated. Building an encouraging group of people is a continuous interaction, yet it's definitely worth the work.

At last, viewing significance and reason in your life can be an incredible asset for adapting to the social shame of diabetes. This can appear to be unique for everybody, except it could incorporate chipping in, associating with your local area, or chasing after your leisure activities and interests.

At the point when you see significance and reason in your life, you feel more satisfied and content. This can assist you with feeling not so much pushed but rather more in charge of your life. Significance and reason can likewise assist you with adapting to the high points and low points of living with diabetes.

One method for seeing importance and intention is to zero in on the things you're thankful for. Appreciation has been displayed to decidedly affect both physical and psychological well-being.

A day to day appreciation practice can assist you with valuing the beneficial things in your day to day existence, even in troublesome conditions.

You can rehearse appreciation by writing in an appreciation diary, saying an everyday petition, or just taking a couple of seconds to consider the things you're grateful for. Indeed, even little things, similar to a decent feast or a warm shower, can be wellsprings of appreciation.

Notwithstanding appreciation, rehearsing self-sympathy can likewise be useful in adapting to the social disgrace of diabetes. Self-empathy implies being benevolent and understanding towards yourself, as opposed to being unforgiving or basic.

This doesn't mean disregarding your slip-ups or issues; however it implies moving toward them with thoughtfulness and care. At the point when you're humane towards yourself, you're better ready to adapt to tough spots and feelings. Self-sympathy can likewise expand your flexibility and further develop your general prosperity.

Once in a while, notwithstanding our earnest attempts, the social disgrace of diabetes can in any case get us down. Assuming you're feeling overpowered or sad, it means a lot to connect for help. This could mean conversing with a confidant in a companion or relative, or contacting an emotional well-being proficient.

There's no disgrace in requesting help - it's an indication of solidarity. Keep in mind; everybody needs support once in a while. Assuming you're battling with your emotional well-being, there's a compelling reason you need to experience it peacefully. Help is accessible, and you have the right to feel quite a bit improved.

As well as connecting for help, it's likewise critical to ensure you're dealing with your actual wellbeing. This incorporates getting sufficient rest, eating a solid eating regimen, and getting customary activity.

Dealing with your actual wellbeing can emphatically affect your emotional well-being. While you're feeling your best genuinely, you're better ready to adapt to the social shame of diabetes. Dealing with your body is a demonstration of taking care of oneself, and it's similarly essentially as significant as dealing with your psyche.

One more significant piece of adapting to the social disgrace of diabetes is defining limits. This implies figuring out how to say "no" to things that don't serve you, and safeguarding your significant investment. It may very well be not difficult to feel compelled to do things you would rather not do, or to over commit yourself.

Yet, focusing on your own needs is significant. This could mean expressing no specific social commitment, carving out margin for yourself, or drawing certain lines on how much time you spend really focusing on others. Limits can be challenging to set, yet they're fundamental for your prosperity.

At long last, commending your victories, regardless of how small is significant. This can be challenging to do while you're confronting the social shame of diabetes, however perceiving your achievements is significant.

Praising your successes, huge or little, can assist you with remaining inspired and positive. It can likewise assist with moving your concentration based on the thing you're missing to what you've achieved.

Have a go at keeping a rundown of your achievements, so you can think back on them while you're feeling deterred. Perceiving your assets and triumphs is a significant piece of adapting to the social disgrace of diabetes.

As well as commending your victories, it's likewise essential to give yourself elegance. This implies being benevolent to yourself when you commit errors, and excusing yourself for not being awesome. Everybody has their faults, and that is fine.

It's critical to gain from your errors, but on the other hand it means a lot to continue on and not harp on them. Keep in mind; you're doing all that can be expected, and that is all anybody can request from you. At the point when you give yourself effortlessness, you'll be better ready to adapt to the social shame of diabetes.

The last way to cope with the social shame of diabetes is to discover a feeling of direction. This could mean finding a purposeful venture, chasing after an imaginative outlet, or chipping in locally. At the point when you have a feeling of direction, you'll feel more satisfied and less inclined to feel the impacts of social disgrace.

A feeling of direction can likewise assist you with feeling more associated with others and to your general surroundings. Viewing a reason doesn't have to be as muddled - it tends to be essentially as straightforward as setting aside a few minutes for a side interest you appreciate.

While adapting to the social disgrace of diabetes can be testing, it's memorable vital that you're in good company. There are a huge number of individuals all over the planet who are living with diabetes, and there are numerous associations and care groups accessible to help.

Go ahead and connect for help when you want it. By dealing with yourself and discovering a feeling of direction, you can capitalize on your life notwithstanding the difficulties of diabetes. Keep in mind, you're not characterized by your condition - you're far beyond that.

Something final to recall is that you have the ability to switch the account up diabetes. You can be a good example for others by sharing your story and pushing for a more sure portrayal of diabetes in the media and in the public eye.

By shouting out and instructing others, you can assist with diminishing the disgrace and make the world a seriously tolerating place for individuals with diabetes. Try not to underrate the force of your voice - it can have an effect.

Summarize, the way to adapt to the social disgrace of diabetes is to deal with yourself genuinely, inwardly, and intellectually. Discover a feeling of direction, praise your victories, and give yourself elegance.

You're in good company, and you can have an effect. With time, tolerance, and backing, you can flourish in spite of the difficulties of diabetes. Keep in mind, you are far beyond a conclusion - you are an individual with a full and significant life.

Assuming you're keen on studying adapting to the social disgrace of diabetes, there are numerous assets accessible. The American Diabetes Affiliation and the Joslin Diabetes Center both have supportive data on their sites.

You can likewise look at the book "Diabetes and Profound Prosperity: A Useful Manual for Overseeing Pressure and Adapting to Diabetes" by William H. Polonsky, Ph.D., CDE. At long last, there are numerous web-based discussions and care groups where you can interface with other people who comprehend what you're going through.

Chapter Nine
Ways to live Well with Diabetes

There are many ways to live well with diabetes; however we'll turn out probably the main ones.

In the first place, it's pivotal to deal with your glucose levels by following a sound eating routine, being genuinely dynamic, and accepting your prescription as endorsed.

Second, make a point to screen your glucose routinely and converse with your medical services group about any progressions in your levels.

Third, practice pressure decreases procedures like reflection or yoga to assist with dealing with your feelings and lessen your gamble of diabetes-related difficulties.

Fourth, try to get standard tests and screenings for diabetes-related complexities like retinopathy and kidney illness.

Notwithstanding the above mentioned, there are a couple of different tips to remember.

In the first place, focus on rest - getting sufficient rest is vital for your general wellbeing and can assist with keeping your glucose levels stable.

Second, don't hesitate for even a moment to request help when you want it - whether it's from your medical services group or from loved ones.

At last, set aside a few minutes for things that give you pleasure and encourage you - this could be investing energy with friends and family, chasing after a side interest, or going for a stroll outside. Taking care of oneself is fundamental for overseeing diabetes.

One more way to live well with diabetes is to track down ways of adapting to the close to home cost of the condition. Diabetes can be an extremely close to home insight, and it means quite a bit to track down ways of handling and manage those feelings.

One method for doing this is through journaling - recording your contemplations and sentiments can be restorative and assist you with acquiring point of view.

You could likewise consider searching out a diabetes-explicit care group, where you can share your encounters and get support from other people who comprehend what you're going through.

There are likewise a few common sense advances you can take to make living with diabetes a piece more straightforward. For instance, keeping a very much supplied kitchen is critical - having good food varieties close by will go with it more straightforward to pursue nutritious choices with regards to supper time.

Another tip is to keep a diabetes unit with you consistently - this ought to incorporate things like a blood glucose meter, an effective wellspring of sugar (like glucose tablets or gel), and your drug. Having these things close by can give genuine serenity and assist you with being ready for any circumstance.

Another functional tip is to attempt to prepare however much as could be expected. For instance, while going out to eat, look into the café's menu quite a bit early so you can settle on a sound decision. While voyaging, pack bites and prescription in your portable suitcase so you don't need to stress over losing your gear.

What's more, in the event that you will be occupied during the day, pack your diabetes supplies in a helpful spot so you can undoubtedly get to them. These are only a couple of models, however the more you can prepare, the simpler it will be to deal with your diabetes.

Beside the down to earth and close to home parts of residing with diabetes, focusing on your actual environment is additionally significant. A perfect and coordinated home can assist with lessening pressure and make it more straightforward to find the things you want.

It's likewise vital to make an agreeable space for testing your glucose and taking your prescription. Having a committed space for these undertakings can assist you with feeling more coordinated and in charge. Dealing with your actual space is only another method for making living with diabetes somewhat simpler.

At long last, zeroing in on your general wellbeing, in addition to your diabetes is significant. This implies eating a decent eating routine, getting ordinary activity, and getting sufficient rest. Dealing with your general wellbeing won't just further develop your diabetes, yet it will likewise assist you with feeling your best. Living great with diabetes implies dealing with your entire self - the whole self.

By adopting a comprehensive strategy to your wellbeing, you can carry on with a satisfying and solid life.

There's another significant element to consider with regards to living great with diabetes - remaining associated with your encouraging group of people. This could incorporate family, companions, medical care experts, and other people who comprehend what you're going through.

Having individuals to converse with, rest on, and depend on can have a significant effect. Recall, it's about who you converse with, yet the way that you converse with them. Tell the truth and be open about your sentiments, and make it a point to request what you want.

One last useful tidbit - remember to set aside some margin for yourself. Living with diabetes can be demanding and debilitating, so it's essential to enjoy reprieves when you want them.

This could mean requiring a couple of moments to yourself every day to unwind or taking a more drawn out get-away when you can. Anything it is, make a point to cut out some time for yourself - it's not self centred, it's fundamental. Carving out margin for yourself can help you re-energize and feel prepared to assume the difficulties of diabetes the executives.

In synopsis, living great with diabetes is tied in with adopting an all encompassing strategy to your wellbeing and prosperity. This incorporates dealing with your physical, profound, and emotional well-being, as well as your socially encouraging group of people and climate.

Make sure to approach things slowly and carefully, and feel free to request help when you want it. You have this - take it each day in turn, and recall that you're in good company. You can carry on with a full and cheerful existence with diabetes, very much like any other individual.

At long last, it's vital to take note of that each individual's involvement in diabetes is one of a kind. There is no one size-fits-all way to deal with living great with diabetes. What works for one individual may not work for another. The main thing is to find what works for yourself and make it a piece of your everyday daily schedule.

It's additionally essential to remain adaptable and versatile - as your diabetes the executives need to change; your methodology ought to change also. The excursion of living great with diabetes is a long lasting one; however it tends to be a satisfying and compensating one in the event that you require some investment to zero in on your prosperity.

One final recommendation - remember to praise your victories en route. It's not difficult to become involved with the everyday drudgery of overseeing diabetes, yet it's essential to require investment to commend your achievements. This could be anything from hitting a glucose objective to tracking down another recipe that works for you.

Anything it is, celebrate it! These little wins accumulate over the long run and can assist you with remaining inspired and positive.

There's another thing we haven't addressed at this point - living great with diabetes likewise implies having some good times! It's not difficult to become involved with the day to day assignments of diabetes the board, yet vital to set aside opportunities for exercises that give you pleasure.

This could be anything from playing a game to perusing a book to investing energy with companions. Anything it is, ensure you're requiring the investment to do things that satisfy you. Living great with diabetes isn't just about dealing with your condition; it's tied in with carrying on with a satisfying life.

To summarize everything, here are the key action items:

- Construct a strong informal community.

- Deal with your current circumstance to make diabetes the board simpler.

- Remain adaptable and versatile as your necessities change.

Following these means can assist you with live well with diabetes. It's not generally simple, yet it's certainly worth the effort.

Just to emphasize, living great with diabetes is definitely not a one-size-fits-all arrangement. It's critical to find the methodology that turns out best for you. Likewise, remember that living great with diabetes is a long lasting excursion.

There will be highs and lows, however with the right help and taking care of one, you can carry on with a blissful and satisfying life. On the off chance that you at any point feel stuck or like you want more help; contact your medical care group or a diabetes support bunch. They can assist you with refocusing and capitalize on your excursion.

Something last to remember is that living great with diabetes isn't just about you - it's additionally about individuals around you. Your friends and family, companions, and collaborators can all assume a part in assisting you with dealing with your diabetes.

They can offer profound help, assist you with remaining focused with your objectives, and even assist you with tracking down better approaches to make diabetes the executives fun and intriguing. Living great with diabetes is genuinely collaboration. So remember to rest on your emotionally supportive network and let them help you on your excursion.

At long last, it's memorable that living great with diabetes doesn't mean never having a terrible day. There will be days when you feel baffled, overpowered, or even crushed. That is totally typical. Simply recollect that one terrible day doesn't mean you've fizzled - it implies you're human.

Try not to be too severe with yourself, and realize that tomorrow is another day.

With time, you'll find that even the awful days get simpler to manage. So approach it slowly and carefully and realize that you have this!

Now that we've covered a portion of the essentials of living great with diabetes, we should discuss a few explicit everyday issues that may be impacted by the condition. One of the most well-known regions is diet and nourishment.

Individuals with diabetes should be particularly aware of what they eat, as it can significantly affect glucose levels. This doesn't mean you need to surrender all your #1 food varieties - it simply implies tracking down sound ways of appreciating them.

There are a lot of diabetes-accommodating recipes out there that are delightful and congratulations. With a touch of imagination, you can in any case partake in your number one food varieties without forfeiting your wellbeing.

One more region that can be influenced by diabetes is active work. Individuals with diabetes need to track down ways of remaining dynamic, as this can assist with further developing glucose control and generally speaking wellbeing.

This doesn't need to mean going to the rec centre for hours consistently - even modest quantities of development can have a major effect. Strolling, extending, and other low-influence exercises can be in every way useful.

In the event that you don't know where to begin, ask your medical services group for suggestions. They can assist you with finding an action that is appropriate for you. What's more, recollect, each and every piece counts!

One more region to consider is rest. Individuals with diabetes need to focus on getting sufficient rest, as unfortunate rest can really make it harder to control glucose levels. In the event that you're experiencing difficulty dozing, there are a couple of things you can attempt.

To begin with, ensure your room is dim, calm, and cool - these are the best circumstances for rest. Then, attempt to lay out a steady rest timetable and stick to it however much as could reasonably be expected. At long last, keep away from caffeine and screens before sleep time, as these can obstruct rest. In any event, rolling out little improvements can have a major effect.

Notwithstanding diet, actual work, and rest, there are a couple of other way of life factors that can influence individuals with diabetes. One is pressure. Persistent pressure can really prompt higher glucose levels, so it means quite a bit to track down ways of dealing with your pressure.

Certain individuals find that unwinding procedures like profound breathing or reflection can be useful. Others observe that exercise is an extraordinary pressure reliever.

Everything without a doubt revolves around finding what works for yourself and integrating it into your daily schedule. Indeed, even a couple of moments of unwinding a day can have a major effect on your general prosperity.

Finally, we should discuss taking care of ourselves. Individuals with diabetes need to focus on their own prosperity, in any event, when it seems like there's an excessive amount to do. This can mean enjoying reprieves when you really want them, rehearsing care, and setting aside a few minutes for exercises that give you pleasure.

It's not difficult to become involved with the everyday requests of life, yet requiring a couple of moments every day to zero in on you is fundamental. Whether it's a hot shower, a decent book, or a call with a companion, ensure you're dealing with yourself.

Something final to remember is that diabetes doesn't characterize you. Indeed, it's a piece of your life, yet it doesn't need to be your entire character.

You're more than your illness, and you have such a great amount to offer the world. It's memorable that you're more than your diabetes, and you can in any case carry on with a blissful and satisfying life regardless of the difficulties it presents. Try not to let the shame of diabetes keep you down -

In the event that you're actually searching for more data on living great with diabetes, I suggest looking at a portion of the numerous extraordinary assets accessible.

The American Diabetes Affiliation has an abundance of data on their site, as well as a helpline that you can require extra help. You can likewise look at books, articles, and webcasts on the subject. There's no lack of data out there - you simply have to find the assets that turn out best for you.

Chapter Ten
Instructions to Converse with Your Primary care physician About Diabetes

Conversing with your PCP about diabetes can be a piece overwhelming; however it's a significant piece of dealing with the condition. There are a couple of things you can do to make the discussion more straightforward.

In the first place, be ready with any different kinds of feedback you have. Record them in advance so you remember anything. Second, make it a point to request explanation or pose inquiries until you comprehend. It's essential to leave the discussion feeling educated and positive about how you might interpret your condition. At long last, make it a point to advocate for you. Your primary care physician is there to help you, yet you realize your body best.

While conversing with your primary care physician about diabetes, there are a couple of explicit themes you might need to cover. In the first place, make certain to examine your side effects, what they're meaning for your everyday existence, and what medicines you've attempted up to this point. Then, examine your eating regimen, exercise, and rest propensities.

It's additionally critical to discuss any meds you're taking, including non-prescription meds and enhancements. You ought to likewise raise any emotional well-being concerns you have, like pressure, tension, or despondency. At long last, remember to examine your objectives for dealing with your diabetes.

As well as examining these points, there are a couple of different things you can do to capitalize on your arrangement.

In the first place, ensure you're ready to take notes - forgetting significant data at the time can be simple.

Second, ask your primary care physician for composed materials to bring back home so you can allude back to them later.

At long last, make it a point to request a reference to another trained professional in the event that you believe you want extra assistance. For instance, a nutritionist can assist you with your eating regimen, and an emotional wellness expert can assist you with dealing with any pressure or uneasiness you're encountering.

With regards to speaking with your primary care physician about diabetes, it's likewise critical to recollect that you're important for a group. Your primary care physician is there to help you, yet you're the one living with the condition.

You know your body and your life best, so don't hesitate for even a moment to shout out on the off chance that something doesn't feel right. Keep in mind, your PCP is your ally, and they need to assist you with carrying on with a cheerful and sound life.

The more you speak with them, the better they'll have the option to help you.

As well as discussing successfully with your PCP, being a functioning member in your own care is additionally significant. This implies playing a functioning job in dealing with your diabetes, as opposed to just adhering to your primary care physician's directions.

For instance, you can follow your glucose levels, screen your eating regimen and exercise, and ensure you're accepting your meds as recommended. Being a functioning member in your consideration will assist you with feeling more in charge of your condition and provide you with a feeling of strengthening.

One of the main things to recollect while living with diabetes is that it's a deep rooted condition. There will be promising and less promising times and you'll need to make changes after some time.

It's likewise essential to recollect that you're in good company. There are many individuals out there who are going through exactly the same thing you are. Associating with other people who have diabetes can be unbelievably useful and strong. It can likewise be an extraordinary wellspring of data and motivation. So feel free to contact others for help.

I likewise need to make reference to that living with diabetes isn't just about dealing with your condition, yet in addition about carrying on with a full and significant life. This implies setting aside a few minutes for the things you love, seeking after your interests, and investing energy with individuals you care about.

Furthermore, dealing with your psychological and close to home health is significant. This can incorporate things like care, journaling, and treatment. Basically living with diabetes doesn't mean your life needs to stop - it's simply unique. You can in any case have a full and cheerful life, even with this condition.

Another significant highlight note is that diabetes can be truly flighty. Here and there, regardless of how enthusiastically you attempt, your glucose levels might in any case vary. At the point when this occurs, it's vital to remain cool-headed and not get deterred.

Simply center on doing all that can be expected with the data and assets you have. It's likewise critical to recall that you're not a disappointment in the event that your levels don't remain inside the objective reach. There are many variables that can influence glucose levels, and now and again it's essentially beyond your control.

In the event that you're finding it challenging to adapt to the eccentrics of diabetes, you might need to think about working with a diabetes teacher. A diabetes teacher is a medical services proficient person who can assist you with fostering a customized plan for dealing with your condition. They can likewise offer help and assets to assist you with adapting to the promising and less promising times of diabetes.

Working with a diabetes instructor can be unbelievably useful, particularly on the off chance that you're feeling overpowered or worried by your condition.

One more way to live well with diabetes is to carve out opportunities to unwind and de-stress. Stress can significantly affect glucose levels, so it means a lot to track down ways of unwinding and de-stress. This can incorporate things like yoga, reflection, or investing energy in nature.

Unwinding is different for everybody, so find what works for you. Simply make sure to set aside a few minutes for yourself, regardless of whether it's only a couple of moments daily. You'll be shocked at the amount of a distinction it can make in your general prosperity.

One last tip is to track down humour in your circumstance. This might seem like an odd idea, however giggling can really assist with lessening pressure and work on your mind-set.

Giggling has been displayed to have various medical advantages, including diminishing cortisol (a pressure chemical) and expanding endorphins (a vibe decent chemical).

So on the off chance that you can find the humour in your circumstance, it can help you feel improved and adapt to diabetes all the more actually. Simply don't make too much of yourself, and attempt to track down the silver lining in even the most difficult circumstances.

Conclusion

Dear reader, by comprehending and implementing the principles in this book, assuredly, you will make positive transformation and improve your health. Thank you for taken your time to read this book. I hope it has inspired you to make positive changes in your diet and health.

www.ingramcontent.com/pod-product-compliance
Lightning Source LLC
Chambersburg PA
CBHW050812260726
48660CB00004B/1383